Alessandra Merendino

The intestine, our second brain

Alessandra Merendino

The intestine, our second brain

Therapeutic gut wellness with water alone

ScienciaScripts

Imprint

Any brand names and product names mentioned in this book are subject to trademark, brand or patent protection and are trademarks or registered trademarks of their respective holders. The use of brand names, product names, common names, trade names, product descriptions etc. even without a particular marking in this work is in no way to be construed to mean that such names may be regarded as unrestricted in respect of trademark and brand protection legislation and could thus be used by anyone.

Cover image: www.ingimage.com

This book is a translation from the original published under ISBN 978-620-6-72146-8.

Publisher:
Sciencia Scripts
is a trademark of
Dodo Books Indian Ocean Ltd. and OmniScriptum S.R.L publishing group

120 High Road, East Finchley, London, N2 9ED, United Kingdom
Str. Armeneasca 28/1, office 1, Chisinau MD-2012, Republic of Moldova, Europe
Printed at: see last page
ISBN: 978-620-8-13541-6

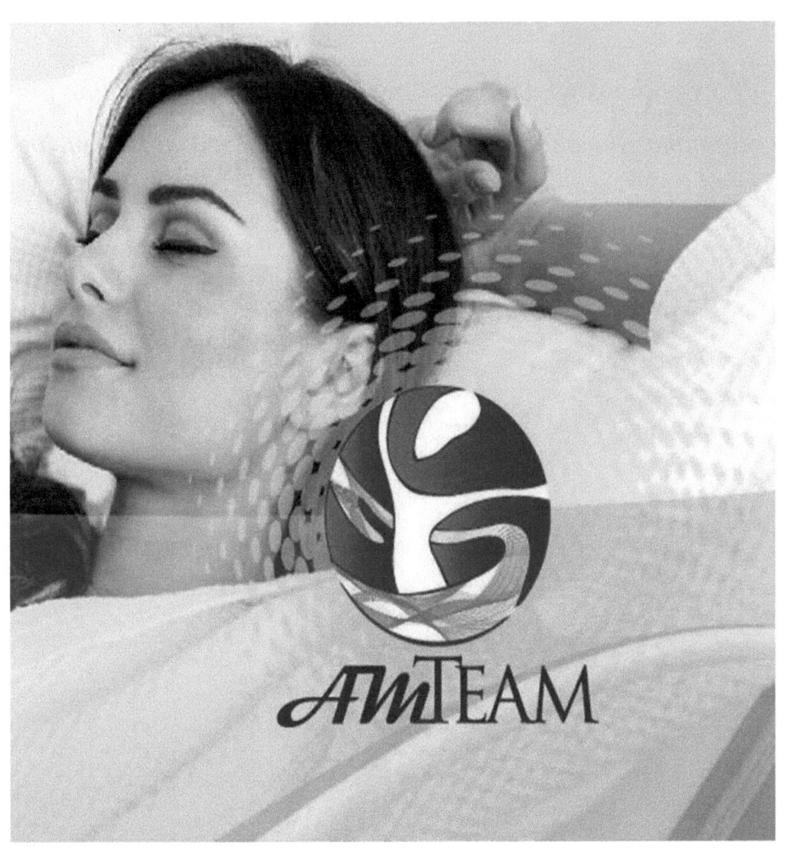
AmTEAM

TABLE OF CONTENTS

MY STORY

My name is Alessandra Merendino and I have twenty years' experience in the field of colon hydrotherapy.

I owe my discovery of colon hydrotherapy to my father, Giorgio Merendino, a doctor who, some forty years ago, while travelling abroad, heard about this therapy. Thinking he could use this method on his patients, he decided to introduce colon hydrotherapy in his medical practice in Rome.

So, during my first year at Rome's 'La Sapienza' University, my training began in this sector and from then on I decided to follow in its footsteps.

I realised that my father's approach to his patients was something special because he was able to turn a medical consultation into a friendly conversation and his smile made people with serious illnesses feel much more at ease.

By following his model, year after year, I have deepened my knowledge and perfected certain aspects of the therapy, transforming hydrocolonic therapy from a medical treatment into a relaxing and enjoyable experience.

In all the doctors' surgeries I've worked in, I've created a special environment characterised by a relaxing atmosphere with background music and a private bathroom.

The first time a patient comes to see me, I explain all the aspects of colon hydrotherapy, any contraindications and have them fill in an informed consent form to agree to the treatment.

I'm convinced that colon hydrotherapy is just the first step on a long journey to better health.

I work alongside many specialists who believe in colon hydrotherapy as a valuable support to their work. Often listening to their patients, they decide to refer them to my practice to have their colon detoxified, seeing this as a first step towards better health. In fact, many medicines are better absorbed by patients when the colon is cleansed of waste: the results of medical treatment are better.

These are the conditions for creating a favourable, win-win situation: for the patients, who are advised by their trusted doctor to begin the journey with this therapy (to really feel better in a relatively short time) and for me, who as a therapist have the opportunity to improve my experience and gather information about particular pathologies and how to contribute to finding a solution.

In my opinion, colon hydrotherapy is just the first step on a long journey to better health.

I work alongside many specialists who believe in colon hydrotherapy as a valuable support to their work. Often listening to their patients, they decide to refer them to my practice to have their colon detoxified, seeing this as a first step towards better health. In fact, many medicines are better absorbed by patients when the colon is cleansed of waste: the results of medical treatment are better.

These are the conditions for creating a favourable, win-win situation: for the patients, who are advised by their trusted doctor to begin the journey with this therapy (to really feel better in a relatively short time) and for me, who as a therapist have the opportunity to improve my experience and gather information about particular pathologies and how to contribute to finding a solution.

Doctors who have an open mind and decide to learn about colon hydrotherapy have the opportunity to achieve better results in less time. In fact, the key lies in cooperation between doctor and therapist.

Very often, doctors are positively impressed by their patients' feelings after the colon hydrotherapy session and their happiness at the new state of total well-being.

Most drugs can't achieve the same results in such a short space of time and patients, on the other hand, are often tired of going to their doctor just to get a prescription for drugs to treat their conditions. They are looking for more than just a pill, which is often expensive and ineffective, to really improve their health.

MY REFERENCES

In the course of my professional career, I have noticed that many people are oriented towards a holistic approach to their state of health and are well aware of the fact that all our organs are deeply interconnected. Some authors, such as Dr Schultze, Dr Adamski and Dr Giuseppe Carano, see our intestine as a kind of 'second brain' and support the idea that it is closely linked to our general state of health.

The simplistic idea that our most important organs are just the brain and heart is changing: our gut really is the key to our health 70 percent of our immune system resides here.

My professional experience is that patients experience a feeling of well-being, not only because they are eliminating their faecal residues, but also because they feel good about themselves and for various reasons they are well aware that they have embarked on a path to improve their health without medication and they see with their own eyes what was in their intestines.

DEEP INTEGRATED HYDROCOLON THERAPY

Of course, I believe that colon hydrotherapy should only be considered as a first step. More and more patients are aware that health is closely linked to nutrition and that it is important to cleanse the colon, but it is also essential to eliminate all the incorrect eating habits that cause inefficient digestion.

Many of the patients I treat every day are unaware that the digestion process begins inside their mouths. They often have very little time to devote to their meals because they have to get back to work, and for this reason the chewing phase is neglected. They generally introduce industrially processed foods into their mouths by chewing them for a short time and then swallowing them. Instead, I suggest that they chew their food slowly several times, mentally counting at least 30 seconds before swallowing. The result is a lighter load for the stomach and, of course, the intestine. It's a simple but effective suggestion.

Another important aspect is prevention. In Italy, the Ministry of Health and many doctors spend a great deal of money encouraging prevention; for an even more effective therapeutic effect, the use of colon hydrotherapy should be recommended to all patients with specific risk factors. In fact, good nutrition and colon cleansing are the best ways of maintaining colon health and reducing the risk of cancer. That's why I work with so many doctors.

When a patient is advised by their doctor to undergo colon hydrotherapy as a preventative measure, it's easier for me to explain all aspects of the therapy and ensure that the patient simply comes back to keep the colon clean throughout the year. The combination of good nutrition and colon hydrotherapy can guarantee excellent results.

MEDICAL-PATIENT-THERAPIST EMPATHY

I would now like to talk about an important aspect: empathy. People often refuse to talk about problems related to their intestines or stools, ignoring problems related to defecation or digestion, and their modesty keeps them away from a practice that necessarily begins with the rectum.

For men in particular, inserting a light into the anus has an impact on their male pride.

The most important thing is to put the patient at ease by making them understand that, in fact, the only thing used for intestinal cleansing is purified water at body temperature.

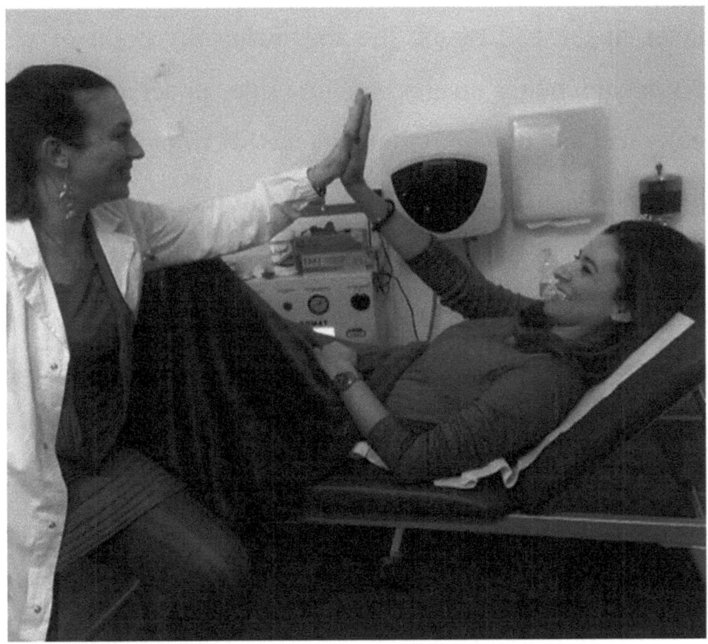

HYDROCOLON THERAPY AS PSYCHOTHERAPY

Hidden, untreated internal problems manifest themselves as stiffness in the tissues, including the intestines. With colon hydrotherapy, we are able to dissolve these hardenings, so that the psychosomatic problem disappears. We therapists only act as intermediaries between what the patient is complaining about, i.e. their real inner discomfort, which stems from their suffering state of mind, the emotionality contained within and what all this generates in their physical, mental and psychological disorder.

The slight discomfort that patients may feel at the beginning is more than compensated for by the feeling of well-being they will experience at the end of the therapy. From my point of view, empathy means being on the patient's side, understanding how they really feel and how important the well-being of the body as a whole is to them.

I often see women of all ages with troublesome inflammations: candida, recurrent cystitis, severe pain in the genital tract, making sexual intercourse difficult. For these young women, it's essential to give them the opportunity to combine the therapy recommended by their gynaecologists, perhaps based on natural products, with hydro-colon therapy sessions that can restore the correct balance of bacterial flora.

They will understand that it will take longer to recover from their illness than with the pharmacological approach, but that restoring balance to their body will also mean less frequent relapses.

A similar problem is faced by all those who suffer from chronic constipation, including, unfortunately, children. One of the approaches most commonly used by doctors is to administer laxatives, which has the effect of trapping them in a vicious circle: they end up becoming dependent on this type of medication and their intestines become increasingly lazy. They will begin to believe that the only way for them to carry out their physiological functions normally is to take purgatives, completely ignoring the ingestion of fibre and physical activity as the most logical and natural solutions.

Sometimes, for this type of pathology, it's easier to prescribe a drug than to resolve the situation more effectively, even if in fact it's often all down to the patient's lifestyle.

Of course, colon hydrotherapy can help to improve their constipation problems, but the best advice is to change the type of diet and physical activity, especially for children who tend to eat only industrially produced foods and spend most of their time in front of a computer or the television.

In such cases, the best thing to do is to talk openly with their parents, who often display similar behaviour in everyday life. These teenagers may also need psychological support.

The idea is that they are (in fact) what they eat.

To do this, it is useful to seek the advice and collaboration of child psychologists who are very familiar with the problems and are able to help people understand the right way to change their lifestyle.

In fact, it makes no sense to cleanse the intestines of a person who, after the first few sessions, continues to live in the same way, chewing rapidly and with little or no physical activity.

To really be on the patient's side, we need to try and understand why they do what they do during the day and what keeps them from a healthier lifestyle. Real prevention consists of avoiding, day after day, the behaviours that increase the risk factors for the most serious diseases. In other words, prevention is not about early diagnosis, but about teaching patients to adopt behaviours that contribute to better health.

NATURAL RIFICATION OF THE BODY

Integrated hydrocolon therapy with visceral massage, lumbar release and insertion of probiotics and natural products, foot and palm reflexology

Hydrocodone Therapy is an ancient medical treatment for the natural purification of the whole body, capable of restoring the correct functionality of the colon. A genuine detoxifying therapy, it consists of an intestinal cleansing using a small jet of warm water at body temperature and low pressure. Colon hydrotherapy completely eliminates the waste that adheres to and has accumulated over the years from the intestinal walls, restoring and reactivating the normal functionality of the colon's mucous membrane and its vital processes.The alternating inflow and outflow of hot and cold water results in faster evacuation. A deeper emptying of the hardest faecal residues that have been stagnating in our intestines for years.

Throughout my personal career of growth and twenty years of professional training, after studying abroad and in Italy, I realised that most Idro colon operators carry out treatment too mechanically without any difference between one patient and another, they do this work to supplement their income without putting any passion or love into it. Instead, I always took each patient to heart, listening to each of their stories rather than clinical, emotional and internal, I realised I had to do more for each of them. I collected all their requests about how this treatment could be done in an environment they considered ideal and their one and only common response was: "Doctor, you who are so delicate, gentle and professional, the only one capable with your gentleness of putting us at ease, we want a more isolated, more private place to relax more". And that's what I did. In my room dedicated to hydrocolonics, I added chromotherapy, relaxing music, an integrated visceral massage, lumbar relaxation, probiotics, purifying herbal teas and natural products, foot and palm reflexology.

HYDROCOLON MERENDINO THERAPY :

1. VISCERAL MASSAGE :

This is a targeted, deep and specific manipulation, not to be confused with a simple abdominal massage, which I perform on the abdomen to facilitate the emptying of the hardest faecal residues.

2. INSERTION OF PROBIOTICS :

The next step is to insert probiotics and natural herbal teas, through a special bottle connected to the machinery, allowing the immediate release of the toughest faecal residues that reside in our colon.

Their direct action in the colon not only results in faster, more effective benefits, but above all leads to the deep elimination of harmful bacteria, fungi and intestinal parasites.

3. LUMBAR RELEASE :

Lumbar unblocking is a procedure performed on the back to remove all the air and detach the hardest faecal impaction in the upper part of the colon.

4. FOOT AND PALM REFLEXOLOGY :

Reflexology is a technique that uses massage on specific points on the feet, hands and knees to restore balance to the body. It is based on the relationship between the nerve endings present in the reflex zones and the point where the pain is present. Pressure on the reflex zone sends communications to the brain, stimulating it to intervene in the problems encountered by the patient being treated. By going to stimulate the intestines of the feet, hands and knees, during the water-filling phase, the patient obtains a greater sensation of relaxation and, as a result, a more rapid emptying of air and waste is achieved.Reflexology has the important capacity to detoxify the body, freeing us from the toxins and waste that clog up the internal organs and alternate their functions. Imbalances in the body are reflected on the surface by painful points and skin changes in specific areas as a manifestation of inflammation spread throughout the body. So, if just one part of the body starts to malfunction, the whole is affected, causing aches and pains that signal the onset of disease.

THE IMPORTANCE OF HERBAL TEAS IN THE MERENDINO METHOD :

Herbal teas perform the important function of eliminating toxins and purifying the intestine, which is the seat of the immune system.

For the Depurative and Deep Detox course in the Hydro colon, different types of plants are used:

DANDELION: The benefits of dandelion are linked to mild digestive disorders including a feeling of fullness, slow digestion, loss of appetite and flatulence. Flavonoids and, in part, potassium salts are responsible for the diuretic properties of dandelions, which stimulate diuresis by encouraging the elimination of excess fluids. Its use is therefore indicated in cases of mild inflammation of the urinary tract, as an adjuvant in minor urinary disorders.

MALVA: a plant with anti-inflammatory and emollient properties, valuable for the intestines, throat and skin. It is an excellent natural remedy for intestinal inflammation, colic and mild constipation, thanks to its soothing and slightly laxative action, which softens the stools and increases faecal mass, encouraging elimination. Mallow is also widely used for haemorrhoids.

FENNEL: as well as being purifying and digestive, it has the ability to eliminate bloating, is rich in antioxidants, helps reduce the formation of intestinal gas and prevents disorders such as meteorism, flatulence and abdominal bloating.

ARTICHAUT: promotes diuresis and aids digestion. It also has purifying, digestive, antioxidant, anti-rheumatic and antibacterial properties. It is highly effective in detoxifying the liver and kidneys, regulating blood sugar levels, combating free radicals and bad cholesterol, promoting the elimination of toxins from the body, improving circulation, diuresis and digestion, and combating swelling.

MELISSE: with its relaxing action, it is beneficial for all pathologies affecting the gastrointestinal system. It is also highly therapeutic for insomnia, irritable bowel syndrome, gastritis, nausea, vomiting, biliary dyspepsia, headaches, tremors, psychogenic dizziness and tachycardia.

TREATMENT PROCEDURES FOR HYDROCOLON MERENDINO :

At the first appointment, there is a short cognitive interview to analyse and identify the patient's specific problems.

After completing the personal data consent and treatment consent form, the patient receives a disposable kit complete with slippers, towel, toilet seat cover, pants and personal disposable intimate soap, for carrying out the treatment.

How does the treatment work?

The patient is made to sit supine on a table. Water at different temperatures is allowed to flow into the intestine through a plastic tube. Thanks to a connected system, the water and dissolved intestinal contents are conducted through a drainage tube.

Then, with a deep visceral massage, the therapist will treat the problem areas, facilitating the release of the hardest faecal residues, before proceeding with the lumbar release. The colonic hydrotherapy thus achieved provides an intensive, total and deeper cleansing of the large intestine than has ever been possible before.

The dissolving action of the water and the simultaneous hot-cold stimulation (as suggested by Dr Giuseppe Carano) thanks to an additional supply of oxygen in the water provide useful bacteria with nutrition. Colon hydrotherapy does not cause pain or cramps, and is considered by patients to be pleasant and beneficial.

The application of hydrocolonic therapy

This treatment effectively eliminates stagnant stools and putrefied substances from the intestinal walls. This natural cleansing process eliminates symptoms that are directly or indirectly related to intestinal dysfunction.

It is characterised by 3 phases:

a) THE DIAGNOSTIC PHASE: in which the conditions of the subject to be treated and the characteristics of his pathology are ascertained in order to establish the right therapeutic approach for his problem.

b) THE PREPARATORY PHASE: in which we try to change the consistency of the intestinal contents to make it easier to empty the colon.

c) THE WASHING PHASE: this is the central element of the therapy and aims to eliminate all faecal matter from the colon, as well as the dysbiotic bacterial flora and the cough.

TESTIMONIALS FROM PATIENTS TREATED BY ME FOR MAJOR PATHOLOGIES

Paola's story :

"Dear Doctor, I am writing to thank you. In just a few days she has given me back my life after so many years! She has brought the sun back into my life, and now I don't have to stare at her from behind a window! Let me explain. In 2000, I was admitted to hospital with acute pancreatitis. At the time, I didn't even know there was such a thing as pancreatitis, or what painful consequences it entailed. Since then, my days, and therefore my life, have been characterised by nausea, vomiting and severe diaphragmatic bar pain. Hospital admissions were frequent and increasingly frequent. When I wasn't in hospital, I was still ill. I was prescribed Plasil for the vomiting, and Contramal and Buscopan for the pain. In 2007 these symptoms were so intense (I weighed 35kg!!!) that it was decided to have biliopancreatic surgery. The operation failed to resolve the pain symptoms. Alongside Lyrica and Cymbalta. In 2008, I was prescribed oxycodone. That same year, I became diabetic. In the meantime, I'm coping badly, with consequences both for my professional life (I'd become unreliable because I often fell ill, 'shirking' the commitments I'd made) and for my personal life and relationships. These 'pancreatic colics' came on suddenly, knocking me out. So I skipped dinners, concerts, cinema, a day at the beach, friends, I stopped travelling. I've even stopped thinking about it! Going to a place where the hospital couldn't be reached at short notice was out of the question for me. In the meantime, in 2014, when I was admitted to hospital with a gastric haemorrhage, I found a k-lung (yes, I'm lucky!). In short doctor, a life of shit hahaha as this word has become dear to me! good day ... toh ... I don't poo. Nor the one downstairs. And I don't even do it the next day. Now, in the midst of all this confusion of symptoms, I have one certainty and that's that I do poo every morning !!!! In fact, this thing catches me off guard. I don't have much information about it. I google it and find everything!!!! Olive oil, vaseline oil, chopped aloe vera. I try everything except...nothing! In the meantime, I go to my doctor and this time I ask him to visit me, to put "his hands on me" and to look at the routine haematological tests, well he can barely finish the visit because of the pain it causes me, and for the first time in many years, the word COLON is uttered, "you have a problem with your colon", and Movicol suggests it to me.but it doesn't work! In short, nothing comes out! Even with enemas, all I expel is water. In the meantime, more than 10 days have gone by. While I'm surfing, I come across IDROCOLON THERAPY. I read on and in desperation booked my first appointment. I was tense and tired, exhausted! I didn't know what to expect, and I certainly didn't expect all this - all this wonderful well-being! No more aches or nausea ... right away! Yes, I felt a sense of well-being from the very first session and I improved little by little! The aches and pains I was talking about have almost disappeared, there's no more nausea, even the vomiting has gone down, and I've got my appetite back and in a good mood! And it's all natural, it's water, just lukewarm water, nothing but painkillers! This year, after so many years, I was able to plan May 1st with friends, outdoors. Thank you, Doctor! I visited many hospitals (Milan, Verona, Rome) and many professionals. In none of them have I found such simplicity in the doctor-patient relationship. Your smile is already therapeutic. What else would I say to you? Don't lose your humanity, that characteristic of yours that makes you special. Treat them as people with their own stories, not just a diagnosis, not just a pathology with which to classify and schematise them, but as unique and irreplaceable individuals. Have a good life, Doctor".

The story of Désirée :

"HYDROCOLON SAVED MY DAUGHTER'S LIFE

I'm Désirée's mother, and my daughter's experience, and that of the whole family, can be described as a real "ordeal". She's a competitive gymnast, and these constant stomach aches have taken their toll on her life, especially at such a delicate time as adolescence. It all started last year with stubborn constipation, and he was stuck for days on end feeling continually ill. I took my daughter to various doctors to solve the problem. The first gastroenterologist who saw her told me it could be a psychological problem, and prescribed purges to be taken every evening, eight sachets in a litre of water (a dose that would also have an effect on a horse), in his opinion the girl would be unblocked. The treatment was to last at least a month, then gradually reduce the dose. After twenty days, there was no response to the medication, my daughter felt ill and vomited for a whole day. She felt bloated, constipated and put on weight, even though she ate very little, sometimes on an empty stomach. My concern grew and I looked for a doctor who could help my daughter by solving this problem. I saw three other gastroenterologists and the answer was always vague, they couldn't tell me what my daughter was doing, they prescribed enemas and purges which did nothing but aggravate the problem. They also doubted that my daughter had undergone the purges and that she was really constipated. This was the most humiliating thing for my daughter and also for me, according to them I would have wasted money and time going to see leading doctors in this field to make fun of them? One of them told me that Désirée could have a malformation of the colon, but that could only be understood by carrying out a colonoscopy, which should only be done after emptying the colon, which was impossible for my daughter. What's more, when I did some research, I discovered that this malformation, if not diagnosed in time, can lead to death. I took a direct X-ray of the abdomen to check for faecal matter and the reports showed the actual presence of faecal impaction in the first part of the colon, which is obviously blocking the passage. A year ago, I'd already heard about colon hydrotherapy, a colon wash performed with body-temperature water that cleanses the colon of all the waste it contains, but why are all the doctors advising me against it, without giving me a solution? It had become a nightmare, my daughter was getting worse and worse, so despite the doctors' advice to the contrary, I took Désirée to the surgery of Dr Merendino, a hydrocolon therapist, who immediately inspired my confidence in his professionalism and humanity. When my daughter started this therapy, she was so blocked that it took five sessions for her to feel better. She is no longer bloated, she feels light and has lost weight, and has reactivated the peristalsis that she hadn't had for a long time. Dr Merendino took our situation to heart and personally accompanied us to the Polimedical clinic in Frosinone, where she is receiving Dr Giuseppe Paliani, who, without taking any charges, immediately realised that Desirèe resists any type of purging. more twisted colon, called dolichocolon, where the stool can stop in certain places and form faecal impaction, which can only be expelled with hydrocolonic therapy. He prescribed an X-ray in transit time, the reports of which show that after the therapy my daughter is emptying regularly and if necessary she will have to repeat the colon hydrotherapy cyclically with maintenance sessions. Now I can say that the nightmare is finally over, and I can say it out loud. It's been a long and tiring journey, but I've finally found doctors who, with professionalism and sensitivity, have saved my daughter's life, solved her problem and given her back her life and her smile. I thank them sincerely and would advise anyone suffering from constipation to have colon hydrotherapy before the problem gets any worse. My biggest complaint is that if I hadn't tried this therapy before, I would have saved my daughter from a year-long ordeal and avoided spending money on visits and medication. This remedy is little known, it's non-invasive and totally natural, it's the water that cleanses your colon that can help prevent many ailments."

The Grazia story :

"A little over a year ago, my bowels stopped working because of chemotherapy, and I tried everything to no avail. Today I had my first hydrocolon therapy session with Dr Merendino who, as well as being an excellent professional, has given me back the possibility of no longer having my back bent from abdominal pain. It was a minimally invasive and very peaceful experience. As soon as the session was over, I felt lighter, straighter with my back and I finally started breathing more deeply again. Thank you Doctor for getting us back on our feet.

THE INTESTINE IS OUR SECOND BRAIN

The key to stress, anxiety and tension lies in the stomach. Here, in fact, there is a veritable second brain with important functions that reverberate throughout the body, regulating emotions, memories and pleasure.

The intestine functions autonomously, helps to fix memories linked to emotions and plays a fundamental role in signalling joy and pain. In short, the intestine is the seat of a veritable second brain. It is no coincidence that the cells of the intestine produce 95% of serotonin, the neurotransmitter of well-being. The intestine releases serotonin in response to external stimuli such as food, but also sounds or colours and internal inputs: emotions and habits. But the reverse is also true: food and intestinal disorders are linked to mood swings. In short, in the stomach is a brain that assimilates and digests not only food, but also information and emotions from the outside world.

What is the link between the skeletal system and colon pain?

The musculoskeletal system is made up of all the bones, joints and muscles, their action supporting the body and enabling its movements, while the colon is the natural breeding ground for bacteria, whose purpose is to neutralise, avoid and prevent the development of a toxic condition in the colon.

Stubborn constipation

People suffering from stubborn constipation may feel the need to evacuate even every 10 to 12 days, so it's intuitive that stubborn constipation is an extremely dangerous condition because it's so close to intestinal blockage. In fact, people suffering from stubborn constipation have fairly clear symptoms, characterised by severe intestinal swelling, meteorism, faecal incontinence, fissures and haemorrhoids.

Intestinal blockage indicates the presence of a total or partial obstruction within the intestinal lumen, an obstruction of such magnitude that it prevents or hinders the normal transit of digestive products. An intestinal blockage therefore occurs when there is an obstructing element inside the intestine that prevents or slows down the transit of food.

When it is particularly severe, intestinal obstruction represents a medical emergency requiring intervention with appropriate treatment as quickly as possible. Depending on the cause, the intestinal blockage may be mechanical or non-mechanical.

By mechanical intestinal blockage, we mean a physical impediment inside the intestine; by non-mechanical intestinal blockage, we mean an impediment to the passage of digested food due to the loss of coordination between the small intestine and the large intestine (coordination which is fundamental to correct peristalsis).

Moving on to the large intestine (colon, sigma and rectum), the possible causes of mechanical intestinal blockage are :

☐ Severe constipation faecal impaction (coprostasis, in medicine, the term faecal impaction designates a mass of faecal matter with a hard, dry consistency, the evacuation of which is very complex, if not impossible, due to the formation of adhesions on the large intestine;

☐ Ovarian cancer;

☐ Cancer of the descending colon and rectum;

☐ Inflammatory bowel diseases, such as Crohn's disease;

☐ Stenosis (i.e. narrowing) of the colon, resulting from scarring or inflammatory conditions.

COLON HYDROTHERAPY AND CHILDREN

My approach to young patients began two years ago following a 9.30pm phone call from Prof. Denis Cozzi, Director of UOC Paediatric Surgery at the Policlinico Umberto I in Rome. Denis Cozzi, Director of Paediatric Surgery UOC at the Policlinico Umberto I in Rome, who asked me to perform emergency hydrotherapy on his 5-year-old haemophiliac patient, Matteo, who had been suffering from persistent constipation for 15 days. The next day, Matteo's parents took him to my studio; the child came in crying from severe abdominal pain.

We began the treatment, and it was only after the first 10 minutes that very hard faecal impacts began to appear, and Matteo immediately began to feel relief and with his big astonished eyes, he looked at his mother with a happy smile, saying: "it's beautiful, beautiful, I feel light". After the first session, in the days that followed, the child was freed and returned to normal.

Later, again through prof. Cozzi, Giorgia arrived at the surgery, whose mother was keen to describe her daughter's experience of Idrocolon in detail:

"My name is Barbara and I'd like to share my personal story about my daughter's constipation problem, which I was able to resolve thanks to colon hydrotherapy.

My daughter Georgia, only 5 years old, has always had problems with constipation ever since she took off her nappy, and as a mother at first I thought it was a psychological problem and the child's insecurity linked to this, as often happens with other children. The situation always got worse and, as a mother, I did what I thought was the most appropriate, also taking advice from the paediatrician. Helping him psychologically with our company in the bathroom or even using suppositories or glycerine pumps. The situation got worse, becoming chronic constipation. A few months ago, a very pressing episode concerned Giorgia: despite these aids, the young girl was unable to evacuate and so on for the next ten days, because she was afraid to go to the toilet. All this combined with psychological stress and pain for the child, but also for us adults, who suffered seeing the child in these conditions. I took Giorgia to hospital, treated her with sachets and thanks to this the little girl was discharged free. Obviously, as a mother, I was relieved and relaxed because I thought I'd resolved the situation, but after a few more weeks the child still couldn't evacuate and thinking I was helping her I gave her the sachets again. This time the child didn't evacuate and unfortunately the situation lasted about twenty days between hospital visits, suffering for the child (she was swollen, she wasn't eating, she was walking bent over in pain, we didn't know how to help her even after the advice of a head doctor from a well-known Roman hospital, But I'd lost confidence and I was also demoralised, because I'd been in hospital several times and no doctor had ever managed to solve my daughter's problem, so given the urgent situation I didn't give any weight to this person who had been referred to me.Days went by and the little girl didn't come out despite the glycerine sachets and pipettes, and I was told that it wasn't possible to act mechanically on this packed stool that had formed. One day I was in a room waiting to visit a specialist and, talking about this problem, I was again recommended to this aforementioned head doctor. So I decided to contact him because I was really desperate and demoralised and I thought I'd try something new. He put me in touch with Dr A. Merendino, a colon hydrotherapist who has been treating adults and children with colon hydrotherapy for many years. After visiting the child, Dr Merendino, having found the child's abdomen very hard and swollen, recommended this therapy to dissolve and remove the hard piece of faecal matter painlessly. Being a child, the situation was very delicate, so this method could be the most suitable. In fact, thanks to Dr Alessandra Merendino's gentleness and delicacy, the little girl immediately felt a sense of relief after the first phase of emptying, and with a beautiful smile she began to feel her tummy deflate more and finally the piece of faecal matter came out. I'm not here to explain the theory of the method as Dr Merendino herself will do, but I can testify that thanks to this painless mechanical action, my daughter freed herself and even in the days that followed she managed to evacuate and even though a few weeks have gone by she's fine. I would advise everyone, and especially mothers, not to underestimate this method and to seek the help of this doctor as soon as this problem arises in their children."

INTESTINAL OBSTRUCTION IN CHILDREN :

This is a complex syndrome characterised by the cessation of intestinal transit of stools and gas. It can be "Functional", to stop intestinal mobility, or "Mechanical", as an obstacle to intestinal transit.

WHAT ARE THE MOST COMMON FORMS?

The most common forms of intestinal obstruction in children are mechanical.

The most common forms are represented by :

- Intestinal intussusception in children aged 4 to 12 months;
- Strangulated hernia in patients up to 3-4 years old;
- Intestinal volvulus on Meckel's diverticulum in children aged 4 to 12 years;
- Occlusion due to adhesion flange in patients who have already undergone abdominal surgery (for example, as a result of peritonitis.

ATTENTION DEFICIT HYPERACTIVITY DISORDER OR ADHD

Main characteristics of the problem

Attention Deficit Hyperactivity Disorder, or ADHD, is a disorder in the development of self-control. It includes difficulties with attention and concentration, impulse control and activity levels. These problems essentially stem from the child's inability to regulate his or her behaviour in relation to the passage of time, the goals to be achieved and the demands of the environment. It should be noted that ADHD is not a normal growth phase that every child must overcome, nor is it the result of ineffective educational discipline, let alone a problem caused by the child's 'naughtiness'.

ADHD is a real problem, for the individual, the family and the school, and is often an obstacle to achieving personal goals. It is a problem that generates discomfort and stress for parents and teachers, who are unprepared to manage the child's behaviour. Parents are no doubt used to seeing how others react to the hyperactive child's behaviour: at first, strangers tend to ignore the agitated behaviour, the frequent interruptions during adult speech and the violation of common social rules. Faced with repeated displays of a lack of control over the child's behaviour, they themselves try to put a stop to the excessive 'exuberance', failing to do so, they conclude that the child is intentionally rude and destructive. Perhaps parents are also accustomed to the conclusions reached by strangers, such as: "This child's problems are due to the way he has been brought up; there should be more discipline, more limitations and even some nice punishments. His parents are incapable, negligent, excessively tolerant and permissive, and this child is the result of their inefficiency". By reading these few lines, parents will realise that, if on the one hand it is becoming necessary to do something to manage the behaviour of these children, it is also true, on the other hand, that it is becoming urgent to make other adults understand what the true nature of the problem of hyperactivity is. Everyone who interacts with children with ADHD needs to be able to see and understand the reasons for these children's behavioural manifestations, putting aside the absurd and unjustified explanations aimed at accusing and hurting their parents, who are already so worried and stressed by the situation.

The first thing you need to know is whether the child you have in mind actually has Attention Deficit Hyperactivity Disorder (ADHD) or whether he or she is just restless and in a daze. No one other than a specialist (for example, a child psychologist or neuropsychiatrist) should feel entitled to decide whether or not this child has ADHD.

Below and on the website, you will find descriptions of the disorder to provide parents and teachers with a clearer definition of the problem, to help them understand which behaviours need to be reduced and which can only be considered as a variable temperament in the child.

TESTIMONY FROM MOTHER CATIA :

"Danny is 14 years old, in the throes of adolescence, with glowing hormones and an argumentative, outgoing, fussy character. Suffering from intestinal candidiasis due to antibiotic treatment from birth to the age of 2, and at the same time suffering from food intolerances.

The benefits of colon hydrotherapy are undeniable. Danny is calmer, acts more lightly in his day-to-day life, smiles and manages his food intolerances better.

- Alex, aged 10, 2nd of three brothers, impetuous schoolboy, hyperactive, wild, jealous, inattentive.

They need constant attention and confirmation if they are not to feel outnumbered by a society that does not wait for or consider a child's real needs and times.

We asked Alex to carry out a colon hydrotherapy session.

The improvement was seen in a gentler child, the hyperactivity was transformed into alertness, today he pays less attention if there are 2 extra potatoes in his brothers' and sisters' dishes, and school has become an interesting friend.

To this day, Alex carries out preventive hydrocolon therapy at each change of season.

- Nicla is 8 years old, a sunny girl with a tenacious character and unbearable whims.

After a session of colon hydrotherapy, it's more reasonable and certainly much more manageable.

To conclude, I am convinced that not only does hydrocolon therapy bring well-being to our body by reorganising it and cleansing it of all waste, but that the proper functioning of our body has positive effects on the body as a whole, as you can read in my testimonial."

WHAT DIFFERENTIATES THE MERENDINO METHOD APPROACH

Colon hydrotherapy is a very delicate treatment and based on my personal experience and my method of treating patients, over the years I've come to realise that over and above technical and manual skill, patients have always had a special relationship with me based on the fact that I've always considered and treated them as "friends"; the treatment has never been about performing the examination itself and that's all, but about a pleasant hour full of laughter, happiness and well-being, first internal and then external.

Seeing my smiling, happy and satisfied patients leave the practice, leaving me beautiful dedications from them, always full of affection, esteem and gratitude, has led me to both improve the environment and make it more welcoming and relaxing.

In this hour of treatment, they find the opportunity to disconnect from the outside world, to escape from all their anxieties, worries and inner pain, which they have never had the courage to bring out on a daily basis because of fear, tiredness and accumulated anger.

To find oneself face to face with someone who is 360 degrees dedicated to them, who is there with and for them to find the right solution to their problems, and who already after the first session feels immediately well, light but above all free of all the weight of inner discomfort has meant that my hydrotherapy method is defined by patients as "the magic effect of the Merendino".

BIBLIOGRAPHY

Giuseppe Carano, *"Idrocolonterapia,ripulire l'intestino per migliorare la salute"*.

Norman Walker, *"La salute dell'intestino il colon"*.

Rudy Lanza, Elisabetta Rostagno, *"Il Benessere dell'intestino"*, curarsi e purificarsi con i metodi naturali.

Miguel Angel Almodovar, *"Intestino, secondo cervello"*, le rivoluzionarie scoperte scientifiche sulla microflora intestinale.

Irina Matveikova, *"L'Intestino, secondo cervello"*, un approccio olistico per una buona digestione e un intestino in salute.

BIOGRAPHY

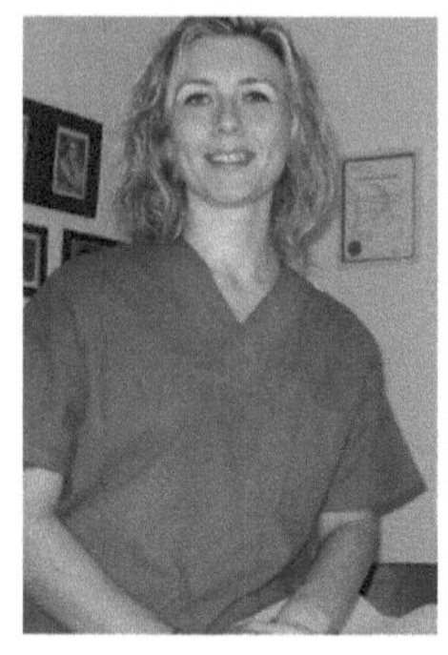 Alessandra Merendino is a colon hydrotherapist and a member of the International Association of Colon Hydro Therapy (I ACT), spearheading a practice that involves the psycho-emotional sphere strictly linked to the functionality of our 'second brain'.

The latest scientific discoveries show just how close the mind-body relationship is, so much so that the intestine has been defined as our 'second brain'. Taking care of it is therefore becoming a fundamental part of our overall well-being.

We can do this simply, with a gentle wash using a jet of warm water, which, without any discomfort, cleanses the colon deeply and effectively, revitalising the whole body and giving it lightness and great energy. The addition of specific probiotics, chosen according to the needs of each patient, recreates optimal intestinal flora.

For almost twenty years, Dr Alessandra Merendino has successfully treated adults, children from the age of 5 and patients suffering from major illnesses such as cystic fibrosis, multiple sclerosis and paraplegia. She is also involved in the preparatory stages of operations on the digestive system.

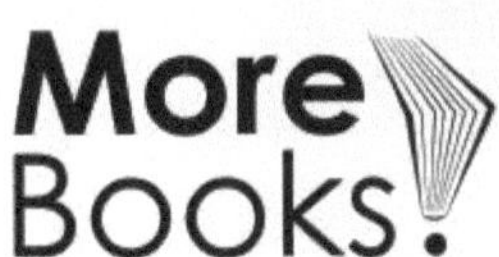

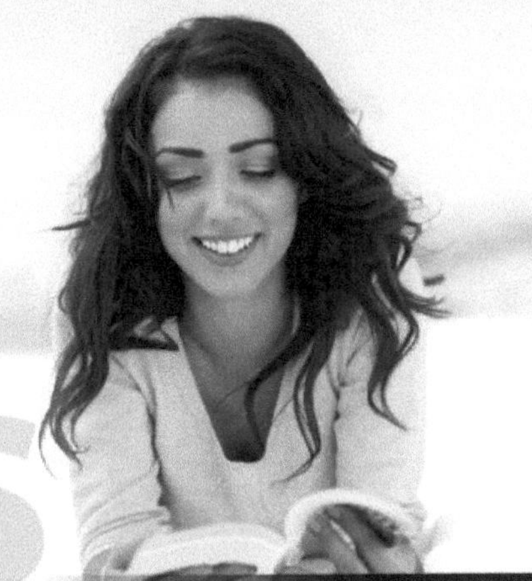

yes
I want morebooks!

Buy your books fast and straightforward online - at one of world's fastest growing online book stores! Environmentally sound due to Print-on-Demand technologies.

Buy your books online at
www.morebooks.shop

Kaufen Sie Ihre Bücher schnell und unkompliziert online – auf einer der am schnellsten wachsenden Buchhandelsplattformen weltweit! Dank Print-On-Demand umwelt- und ressourcenschonend produzi ert.

Bücher schneller online kaufen
www.morebooks.shop

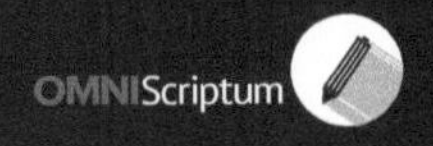

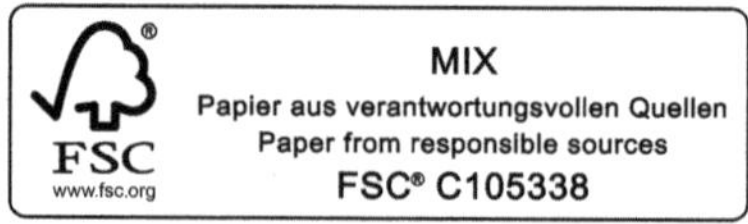

Printed by Books on Demand GmbH, Norderstedt / Germany